WHISPERS OF PARENTHOOD

By:

AROWOLO HABEEB

Table of Contents

Chapter One: Unexpected Encounter

The quaint town of Evercrest bustled with its daily rhythm as Sarah strolled along the cobblestone streets, her eyes fixed on the storefronts adorned with vibrant displays. With a folder clasped tightly under her arm and determination in her stride, she was on a mission—the pursuit of a job that resonated with her passion for social causes.

As she rounded a corner, she almost collided with a man exiting a towering glass building. Sarah stumbled back, her folder slipping from her grasp, scattering papers across the sidewalk. With a swift reflex, the man reached out, catching some of the fluttering pages mid-air.

"I'm so sorry," Sarah murmured, her cheeks flushed with embarrassment, kneeling to gather the stray papers.

"No harm done," the man replied, a gentle smile gracing his lips. His dark eyes met hers briefly before he crouched down, helping her collect the documents.

Their hands briefly brushed as they reached for the same page, a momentary spark igniting between them—a flash of connection that caught Sarah off guard.

"I'm Sarah," she offered, smiling softly.

"Jackson," he replied, returning her smile. There was an enigmatic allure about him, an air of mystery that piqued Sarah's curiosity.

Their unexpected encounter lingered in Sarah's thoughts as she continued her quest for employment. Little did she know that this serendipitous meeting with Jackson would mark the beginning of an unforeseen chapter in her life.

Chapter Two: Echoes of Loss

Sarah sat by the window of her modest apartment, the fading light casting shadows across the room. She traced the edges of a weathered photograph—an image frozen in time, capturing her childhood with her father, a man whose absence still echoed in her life.

Her father's premature departure left a void that no passage of time could fill. Memories of his warmth, his laughter, and his unwavering support lingered like fragile echoes. He was the beacon of strength in their modest household, raising Sarah single-handedly after her mother passed away when she was a tender age.

Growing up, she witnessed her father's tireless dedication to provide for them, instilling in her the values of resilience and empathy. His absence etched a bittersweet mark on Sarah's life, shaping her into the compassionate and determined individual she had become.

As she flipped through old letters and cherished mementos, memories of her mother's unwavering love and her father's sacrifices flooded her thoughts, reminding her of the foundation upon which she built her aspirations.

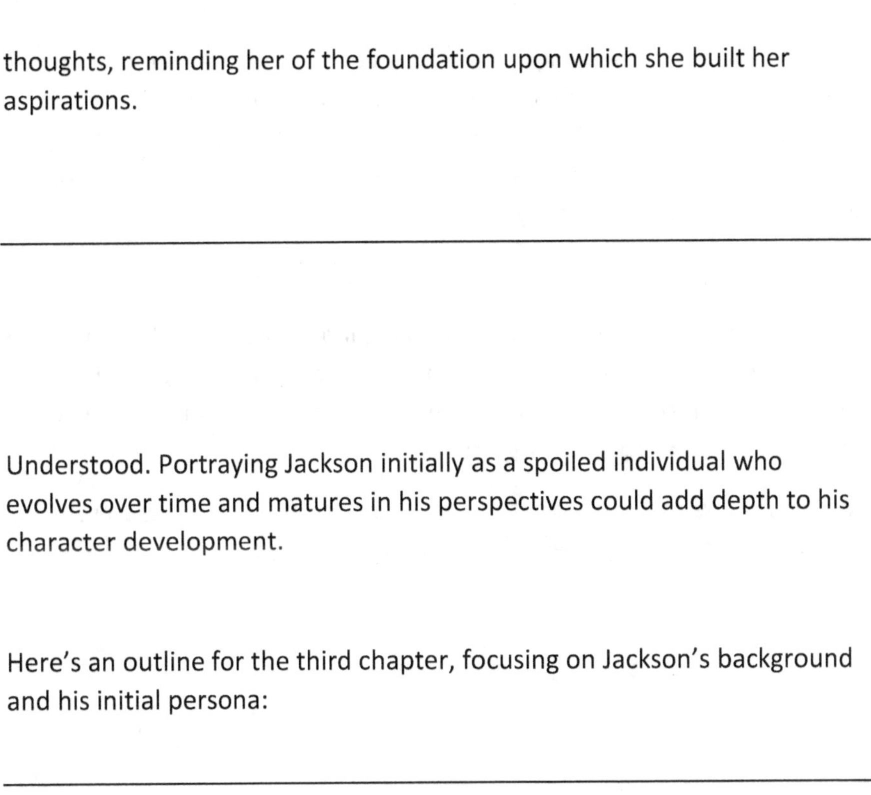

Understood. Portraying Jackson initially as a spoiled individual who evolves over time and matures in his perspectives could add depth to his character development.

Here's an outline for the third chapter, focusing on Jackson's background and his initial persona:

Chapter Three: Shadows of Wealth

In the opulent halls of the lavish estate that housed the Calloway family, Jackson Calloway lounged in the comfort of luxury—a testament to the opulence and wealth that surrounded him since birth.

Raised in the lap of luxury, Jackson was accustomed to a life of privilege and indulgence, shielded from the harsher realities by his family's immense fortune. His carefree demeanor often masked the deeper conflicts that stirred within him, remnants of a past marred by the absence of genuine connections and meaningful relationships.

Adored by many for his charm and affluence, Jackson indulged in a playboy lifestyle, a guise that shielded him from emotional entanglements. His fleeting romances and the string of broken hearts became part of his persona—a man who wielded his wealth and charisma as shields against vulnerability.

Yet, as he matured, the shadows of his past indulgences weighed on his conscience. Echoes of his callous actions lingered, prompting a yearning for something more substantial—a desire for genuine connections that transcended superficial encounters.

Certainly! Jackson's evolution from a playboy persona to a person seeking genuine connections can be a multi-faceted journey.

Chapter Four: Shadows Receding

Amidst the glittering soirées and whispers of his lavish lifestyle, Jackson found himself grappling with a sense of discontent that lingered like a shadow—a silent reminder of his superficial past.

The allure of fleeting romances and casual encounters that once defined his existence now felt hollow, leaving an emptiness that his wealth and charm couldn't fill. Each broken relationship, once a conquest to him, now echoed with a haunting sense of remorse.

A chance encounter with Sarah, her genuine nature and unwavering dedication to her cause, sparked a dormant ember within Jackson—a yearning for something beyond the superficial façade he had cultivated.

As he witnessed Sarah's unyielding determination and witnessed the depth of her compassion, Jackson found himself drawn to her in ways he hadn't experienced before. Her authenticity and genuine nature became a stark contrast to the shallowness that had defined his previous interactions.

Slowly but steadily, Sarah's presence ignited a desire within Jackson for a more meaningful connection, prompting introspection and a gradual shedding of his former playboy persona. His journey towards authenticity and a deeper understanding of love and relationships began to take root, reshaping his outlook on life.

Chapter Five: Awakening Desires

In the tranquil moments of solitude, Jackson found himself haunted by echoes of his past—ghosts of fleeting encounters that once defined his existence. Yet, amidst these shadows, a beacon of light emerged, emanating from the unwavering presence of Sarah in his life.

As their paths intertwined, Jackson's perspective on relationships underwent a profound shift. He found himself captivated by Sarah's authenticity and unwavering dedication—a stark contrast to the shallowness that once dominated his world.

The self-imposed barriers he had erected around his heart began to crumble under the weight of Sarah's genuine nature. Her unassuming demeanor and heartfelt conversations sparked emotions within him that he had long kept dormant—a yearning for connection beyond the superficial.

Each shared moment with Sarah became a revelation, unraveling layers of his persona, stirring emotions he had shielded behind a mask of indifference. Her compassion, dedication, and unwavering principles awakened a desire within him for a depth of connection he had never pursued before.

In Sarah's presence, he discovered a newfound vulnerability—one that compelled him to confront his past actions and seek redemption for the hearts he had callously disregarded. His transformation from a man of superficial conquests to someone yearning for authentic connections became an arduous yet soul-stirring journey.

Chapter Six: Vulnerability Unveiled

Amidst an evening draped in a symphony of stars, Sarah and Jackson found themselves engulfed in a conversation that transcended the realms of casual banter. The soft glow of moonlight bathed their surroundings as they sat under a canopy of twinkling constellations, their exchange of words echoing in the tranquil night.

As Sarah spoke passionately about her dedication to her cause, the earnestness in her voice resonated within Jackson's soul. Her unwavering commitment and compassionate ideals painted a stark contrast to the frivolous encounters he had once embraced.

In the rawness of that moment, Jackson found himself baring his soul in ways he never thought possible. Vulnerability, a facet he had shielded from the world, emerged as he confided in Sarah about his struggles, his past mistakes, and the relentless pursuit of superficial connections.

The weight of his confessions hung in the air, mingling with the gentle breeze. Sarah listened, her empathy and understanding acting as a balm to his wounded spirit. In that vulnerable exchange, Jackson felt a sense of liberation—a departure from the facade he had meticulously crafted.

The warmth of Sarah's acceptance, devoid of judgment, unearthed emotions he had long suppressed. It was in that moment of unguarded honesty that Jackson realized the profound impact Sarah had on him—the catalyst for his transformation, propelling him towards a path of introspection and self-discovery.

Chapter Seven: The Unspoken Bond

In the wake of their vulnerable exchange, an unspoken understanding blossomed between Sarah and Jackson. Their connection, once tethered by shared moments of vulnerability, now expanded into a profound bond—a silent language of unspoken emotions that intertwined their lives.

Sarah's unwavering support and genuine encouragement became an anchor in Jackson's life. Her presence brought solace, a refuge from the superficiality that once clouded his existence. With her, he discovered an unprecedented sense of belonging, a haven he hadn't known he craved.

Their interactions were no longer confined to mere conversations; each glance, each touch, held unspoken sentiments that echoed the depth of their growing affection. Sarah's compassionate nature continued to inspire Jackson, nudging him further along the path of self-discovery and introspection.

Amidst shared moments of laughter and quiet contemplation, their connection flourished, weaving a tapestry of understanding and trust. Each day spent in each other's company further solidified their bond—a bond woven with threads of vulnerability, mutual respect, and an unwavering desire for genuine connection.

Their relationship, once an unexpected encounter, had now evolved into a journey of mutual growth and emotional exploration—a testament to the transformative power of genuine connection and heartfelt understanding.

Chapter Eight: Trials of Trust

As Sarah and Jackson's bond deepened, the echoes of their pasts lingered, casting fleeting shadows on their journey together. Amidst their growing affection, doubts began to surface—a consequence of their contrasting backgrounds and the ghosts they carried from their past.

Sarah, despite her unwavering support, found herself wrestling with moments of insecurity, a remnant of her past experiences. Jackson's affluent upbringing stood in stark contrast to her humble origins, planting seeds of doubt about their compatibility and the acceptance she sought within his world.

Conversely, Jackson grappled with the remnants of his playboy persona, haunted by the misconceptions that colored his reputation. Fearful of being judged by Sarah's unwavering standards, he concealed his insecurities behind a façade, hesitant to reveal the vulnerable truths he had shared earlier.

Their unspoken fears and hesitations created a subtle strain in their otherwise burgeoning relationship. Misunderstandings and moments of hesitance became a subtle barrier, clouding the once-clear skies of their budding romance.

Yet, amidst the trials of trust, Sarah and Jackson found solace in the depth of their connection. Their commitment to understanding each other's vulnerabilities and fears became the catalyst for navigating the stormy seas of doubt—a testament to their resilience and determination to weather the challenges together.

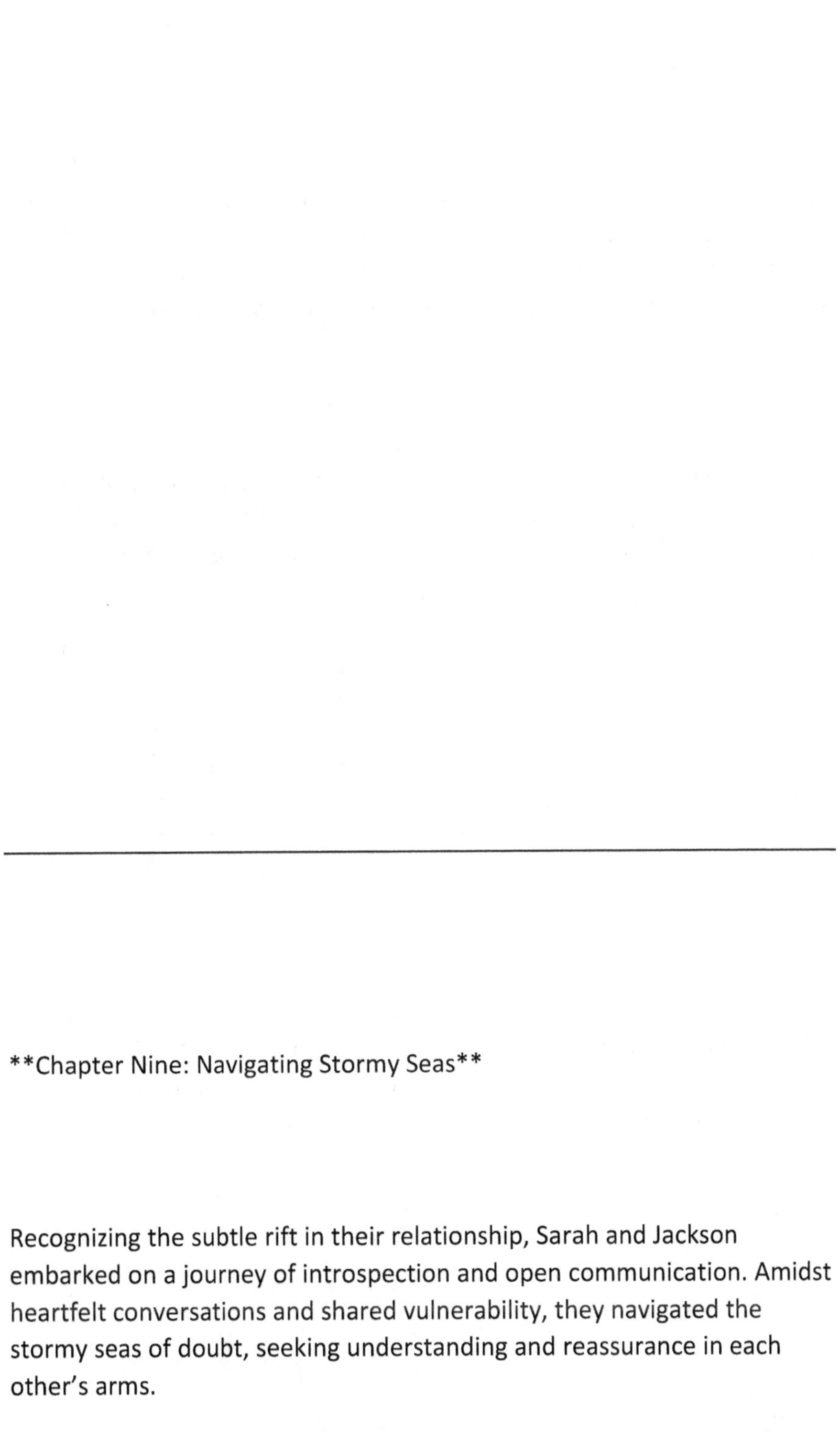

Chapter Nine: Navigating Stormy Seas

Recognizing the subtle rift in their relationship, Sarah and Jackson embarked on a journey of introspection and open communication. Amidst heartfelt conversations and shared vulnerability, they navigated the stormy seas of doubt, seeking understanding and reassurance in each other's arms.

Sarah, with her unwavering empathy, extended a hand of understanding, reassuring Jackson of her acceptance and appreciation for the person he had become. Her genuine affection and unconditional support became an anchor in his turbulent seas, eroding the walls of his self-doubt.

In turn, Jackson shed the veneer of indifference, baring his insecurities and fears to Sarah, revealing the vulnerable truths he had long concealed. His honesty and willingness to confront his past allowed Sarah to see the depth of his transformation and genuine desire for their relationship.

Their open and heartfelt conversations fostered an environment of trust and understanding. Each shared moment became an opportunity for healing and growth, a testament to their resilience and commitment to each other.

Through mutual empathy and unwavering support, Sarah and Jackson emerged from the tempest stronger than before—a testament to the transformative power of open communication and genuine connection.

Chapter Ten: Embracing New Horizons

As the tempest of doubts receded, Sarah and Jackson emerged stronger, their bond fortified by the trials they had weathered together. Their relationship entered a new phase—an era marked by a deeper understanding and unwavering commitment to each other.

With newfound clarity and a shared vision, Sarah and Jackson embarked on a journey of exploration and shared experiences. They embraced each moment with a fervor, cherishing the simple joys and celebrating milestones that marked their path.

Their shared adventures, from spontaneous escapades in bustling cities to tranquil retreats in serene landscapes, became cherished memories etched in the canvas of their budding romance. Amidst laughter, shared dreams, and whispered promises, they forged a path paved with mutual respect and unwavering support.

In the quietude of intimate moments and the exuberance of shared passions, Sarah and Jackson found solace—a sanctuary within each other's presence. Their relationship had transformed into a sanctuary where vulnerability was celebrated, and love blossomed in its purest form.

Their journey together, once marked by uncertainties and trials, had now evolved into a harmonious symphony—a testament to the transformative power of trust, understanding, and genuine affection.

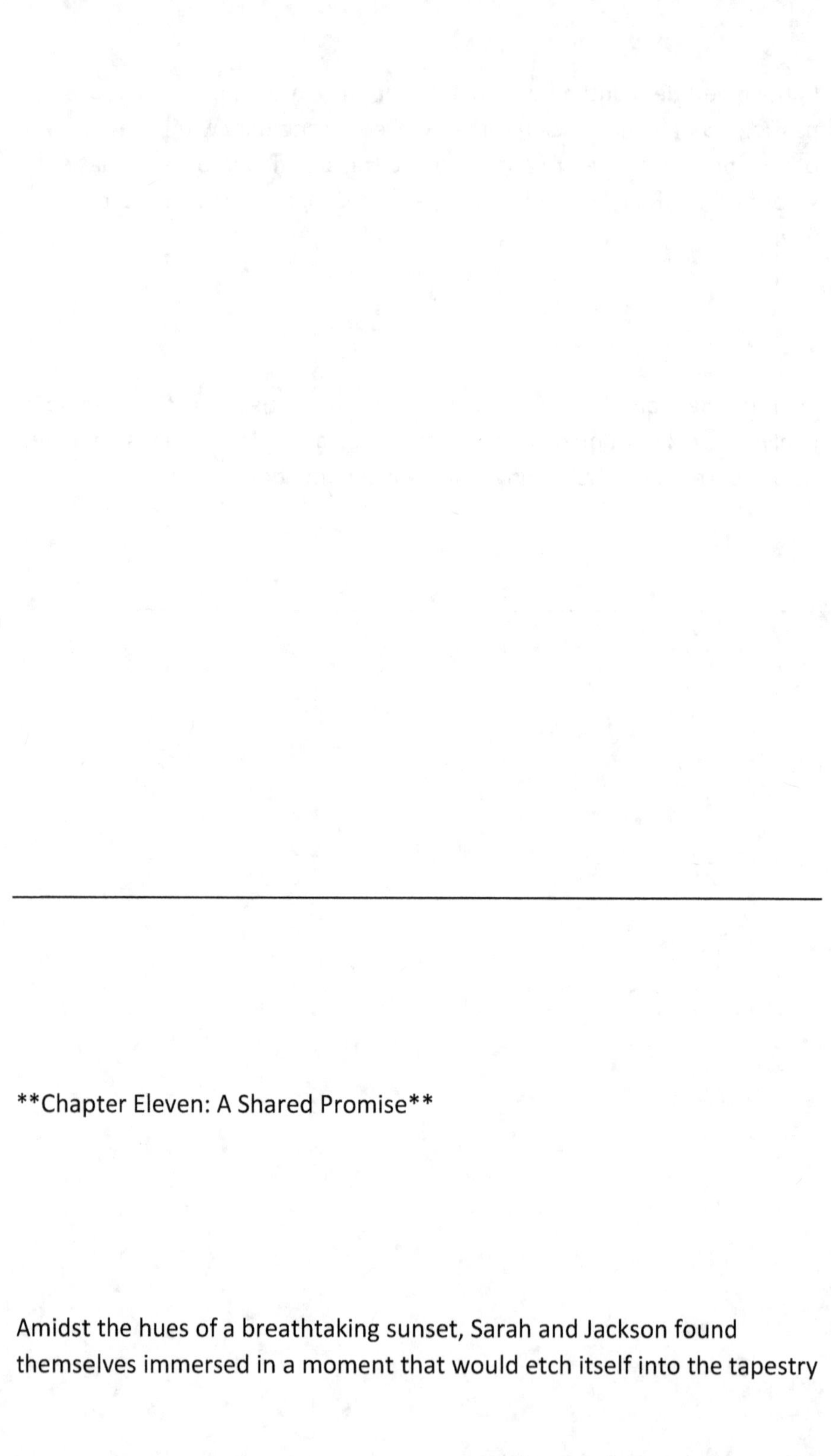

Chapter Eleven: A Shared Promise

Amidst the hues of a breathtaking sunset, Sarah and Jackson found themselves immersed in a moment that would etch itself into the tapestry of their lives—a moment woven with anticipation and an unwavering commitment to each other.

In the tranquil serenity of a picturesque garden, surrounded by fragrant blossoms and the soft melody of nature, Jackson knelt before Sarah, a glimmer of nervous excitement dancing in his eyes.

With a trembling yet earnest voice, he spoke words that echoed with the depth of his affection and the sincerity of his heart—a declaration of love and an unwavering promise to stand by her side through life's ebbs and flows.

Tears welled in Sarah's eyes as she gazed into the eyes of the man she had grown to love—a man whose transformation had touched her soul in ways she never thought possible. Her trembling voice reciprocated his heartfelt sentiments, sealing their bond with promises of unwavering support and endless devotion.

In that moment, amidst the golden hues of twilight, Sarah and Jackson embraced their shared promise—a testament to their journey, their growth, and the depth of their enduring love.

Chapter Twelve: Uncharted Paths

With their shared promise nestled within their hearts, Sarah and Jackson embarked on a new chapter—a chapter illuminated by the warmth of their love and the anticipation of an intertwined future.

Their days were painted with hues of shared dreams and mutual aspirations. Sarah's unwavering dedication to her cause continued to inspire Jackson, spurring him to explore avenues where his privilege could be a force for positive change.

As they navigated life's uncharted paths, Sarah's resilience and Jackson's newfound purpose created a harmonious synergy—a partnership built on mutual respect and unwavering support. Their relationship became a haven where they found solace amidst life's complexities.

Through triumphs and challenges, they remained steadfast in their commitment, celebrating each other's victories and offering unwavering support during moments of adversity. Their shared promise acted as a guiding beacon, illuminating the unknown paths they traversed together.

Amidst shared laughter, whispered confessions, and the gentle rhythm of their intertwined lives, Sarah and Jackson forged ahead—a testament to the enduring strength of their love and the depth of their unspoken bondW

Chapter Thirteen: Building Dreams

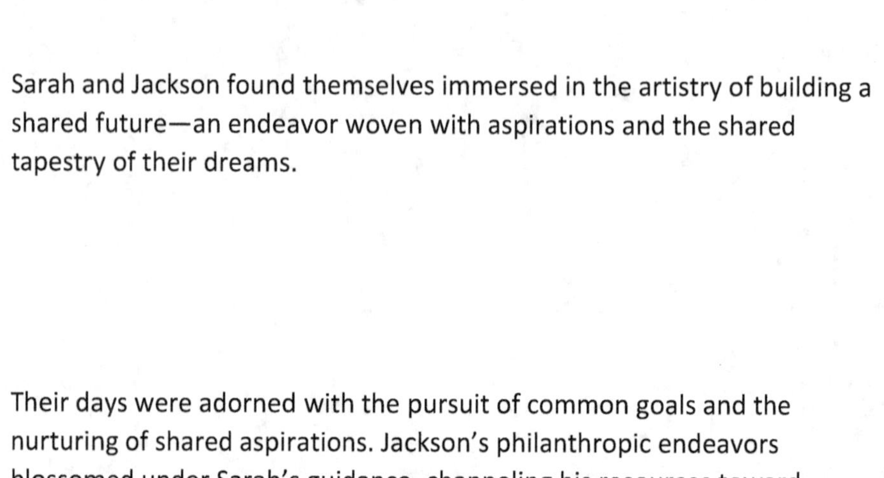

Sarah and Jackson found themselves immersed in the artistry of building a shared future—an endeavor woven with aspirations and the shared tapestry of their dreams.

Their days were adorned with the pursuit of common goals and the nurturing of shared aspirations. Jackson's philanthropic endeavors blossomed under Sarah's guidance, channeling his resources toward causes close to both their hearts.

Together, they carved a sanctuary within their home—a haven that echoed with shared laughter and whispered promises. Each nook and corner bore traces of their individual personalities, seamlessly blending into a harmonious space they called their own.

In the sanctuary of their shared abode, they embarked on new adventures—culinary escapades that mirrored their diverse tastes, quiet evenings spent lost in the pages of cherished books, and moments of shared creativity that breathed life into their shared passions.

Their life together became a canvas painted with hues of companionship and mutual understanding—a testament to their commitment to building a future steeped in love, respect, and shared endeavors.

Chapter Fourteen: Nurturing Bonds

As their journey unfolded, Sarah and Jackson found themselves immersed in the artistry of nurturing bonds beyond their own. Their shared commitment to their relationship extended to fostering connections with those around them.

Their home became a gathering place—a sanctuary where friends, old and new, found solace amidst the warmth of their companionship. Each gathering echoed with laughter and heartfelt conversations, weaving a web of cherished relationships.

In the realm of their shared existence, Sarah and Jackson found themselves extending their compassion beyond their immediate circle. Their dedication to philanthropy bore fruit in endeavors that reached out to the community, leaving an indelible mark of positive change.

Amidst their shared commitments, they discovered a mutual passion for advocacy—standing shoulder to shoulder in support of causes that echoed their shared values. Their unified voice became a beacon, advocating for positive change and fostering a ripple effect of compassion and understanding.

Their shared efforts, rooted in a foundation of empathy and genuine concern, showcased the depth of their bond and their unwavering commitment to making a meaningful impact in the lives of those around them.

Chapter Fifteen: Embracing Change

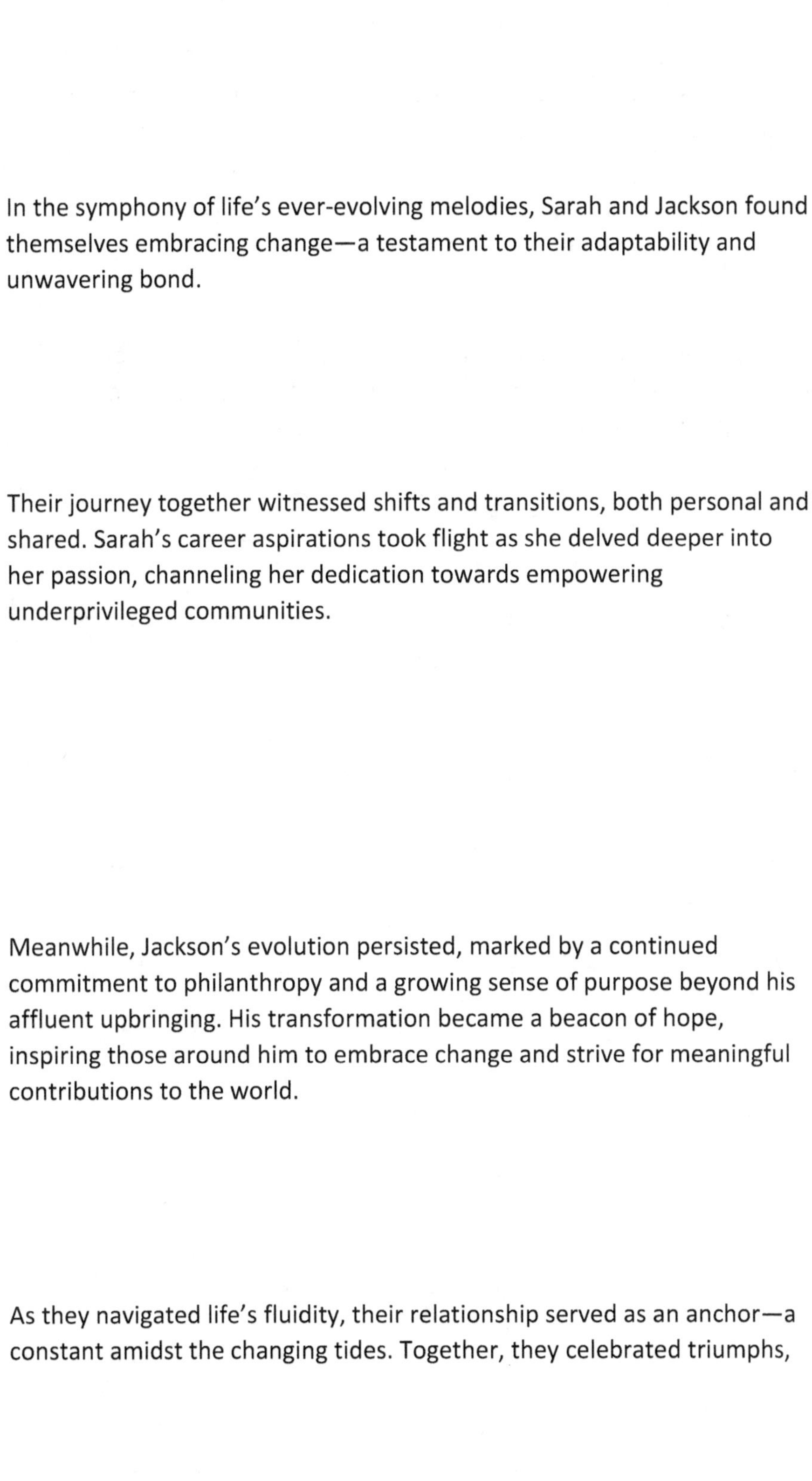

In the symphony of life's ever-evolving melodies, Sarah and Jackson found themselves embracing change—a testament to their adaptability and unwavering bond.

Their journey together witnessed shifts and transitions, both personal and shared. Sarah's career aspirations took flight as she delved deeper into her passion, channeling her dedication towards empowering underprivileged communities.

Meanwhile, Jackson's evolution persisted, marked by a continued commitment to philanthropy and a growing sense of purpose beyond his affluent upbringing. His transformation became a beacon of hope, inspiring those around him to embrace change and strive for meaningful contributions to the world.

As they navigated life's fluidity, their relationship served as an anchor—a constant amidst the changing tides. Together, they celebrated triumphs, weathered storms, and found solace in the unwavering support they offered each other.

Their journey together became a testament to the beauty of evolution—a tapestry woven with threads of growth, shared values, and an enduring love that remained unshaken amidst life's myriad transitions.

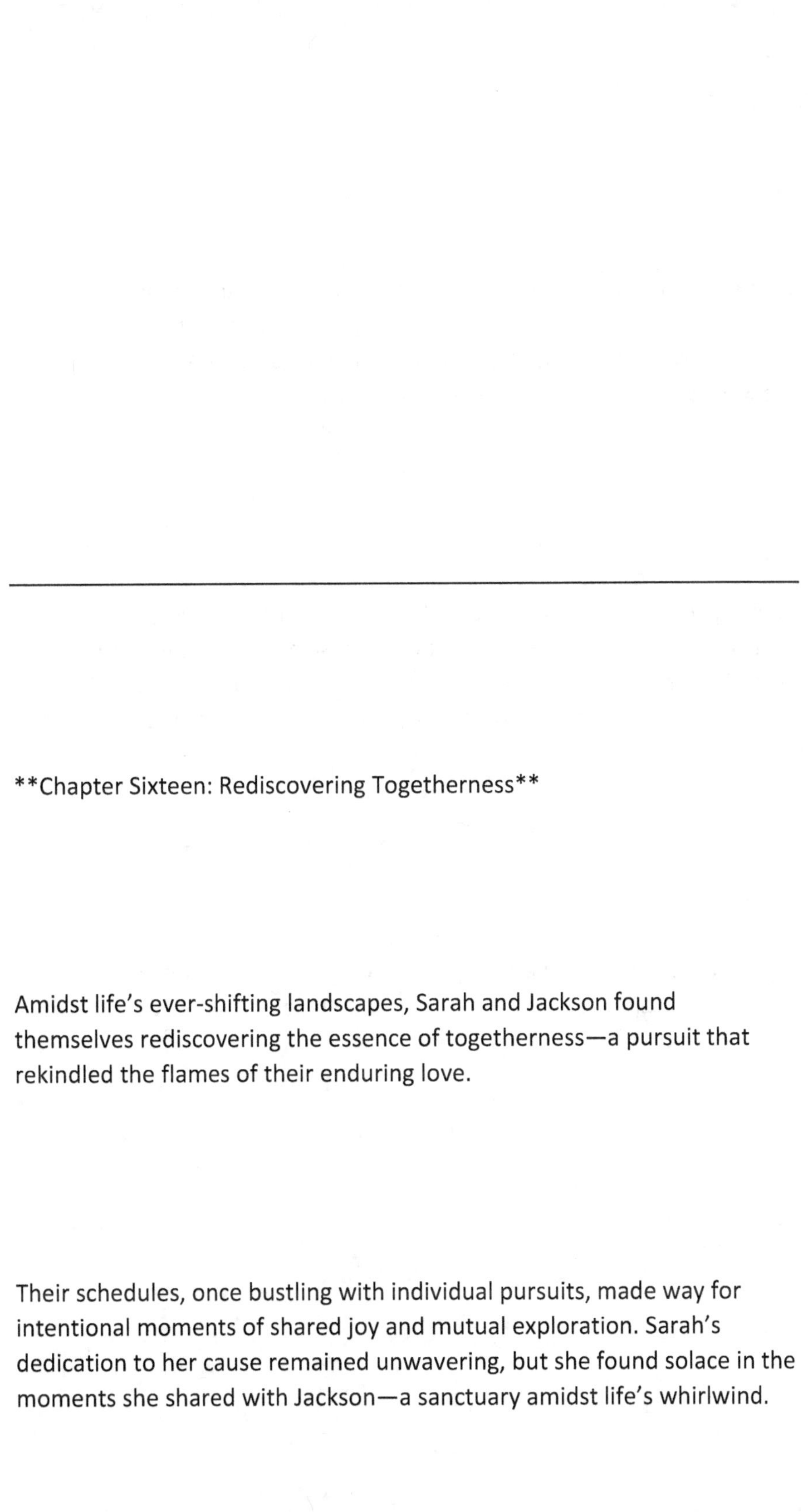

Chapter Sixteen: Rediscovering Togetherness

Amidst life's ever-shifting landscapes, Sarah and Jackson found themselves rediscovering the essence of togetherness—a pursuit that rekindled the flames of their enduring love.

Their schedules, once bustling with individual pursuits, made way for intentional moments of shared joy and mutual exploration. Sarah's dedication to her cause remained unwavering, but she found solace in the moments she shared with Jackson—a sanctuary amidst life's whirlwind.

Conversely, Jackson's philanthropic endeavors continued to flourish, but he carved deliberate spaces in his life to nurture their relationship. Moments of quiet intimacy and shared passions became a cherished respite from the demands of their respective journeys.

Their bond, weathered by time and fortified by shared experiences, blossomed anew—an embodiment of the resilience and unwavering commitment they held for each other. In the ebb and flow of life, they discovered the beauty of balancing individual growth with the nurturing of their relationship.

Their journey of rediscovery served as a testament to the enduring strength of their love—a love that remained steadfast amidst the evolving chapters of their lives.

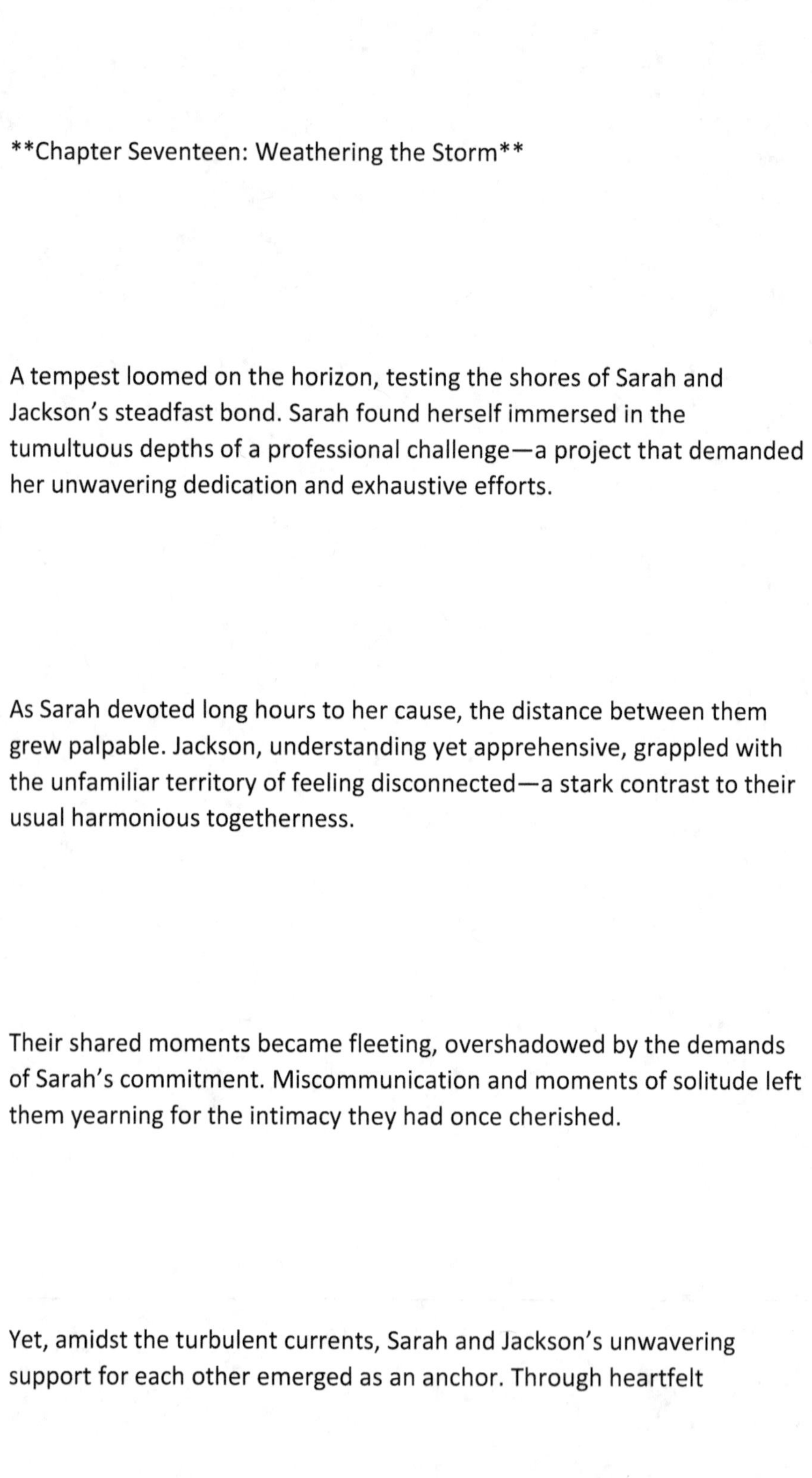

Chapter Seventeen: Weathering the Storm

A tempest loomed on the horizon, testing the shores of Sarah and Jackson's steadfast bond. Sarah found herself immersed in the tumultuous depths of a professional challenge—a project that demanded her unwavering dedication and exhaustive efforts.

As Sarah devoted long hours to her cause, the distance between them grew palpable. Jackson, understanding yet apprehensive, grappled with the unfamiliar territory of feeling disconnected—a stark contrast to their usual harmonious togetherness.

Their shared moments became fleeting, overshadowed by the demands of Sarah's commitment. Miscommunication and moments of solitude left them yearning for the intimacy they had once cherished.

Yet, amidst the turbulent currents, Sarah and Jackson's unwavering support for each other emerged as an anchor. Through heartfelt conversations and deliberate efforts, they bridged the emotional chasm that threatened their bond.

Their commitment to understanding and empathy acted as a salve, healing the wounds of distance. With patience and mutual reassurance, they navigated the storm, emerging stronger, their bond fortified by the trials they weathered together.

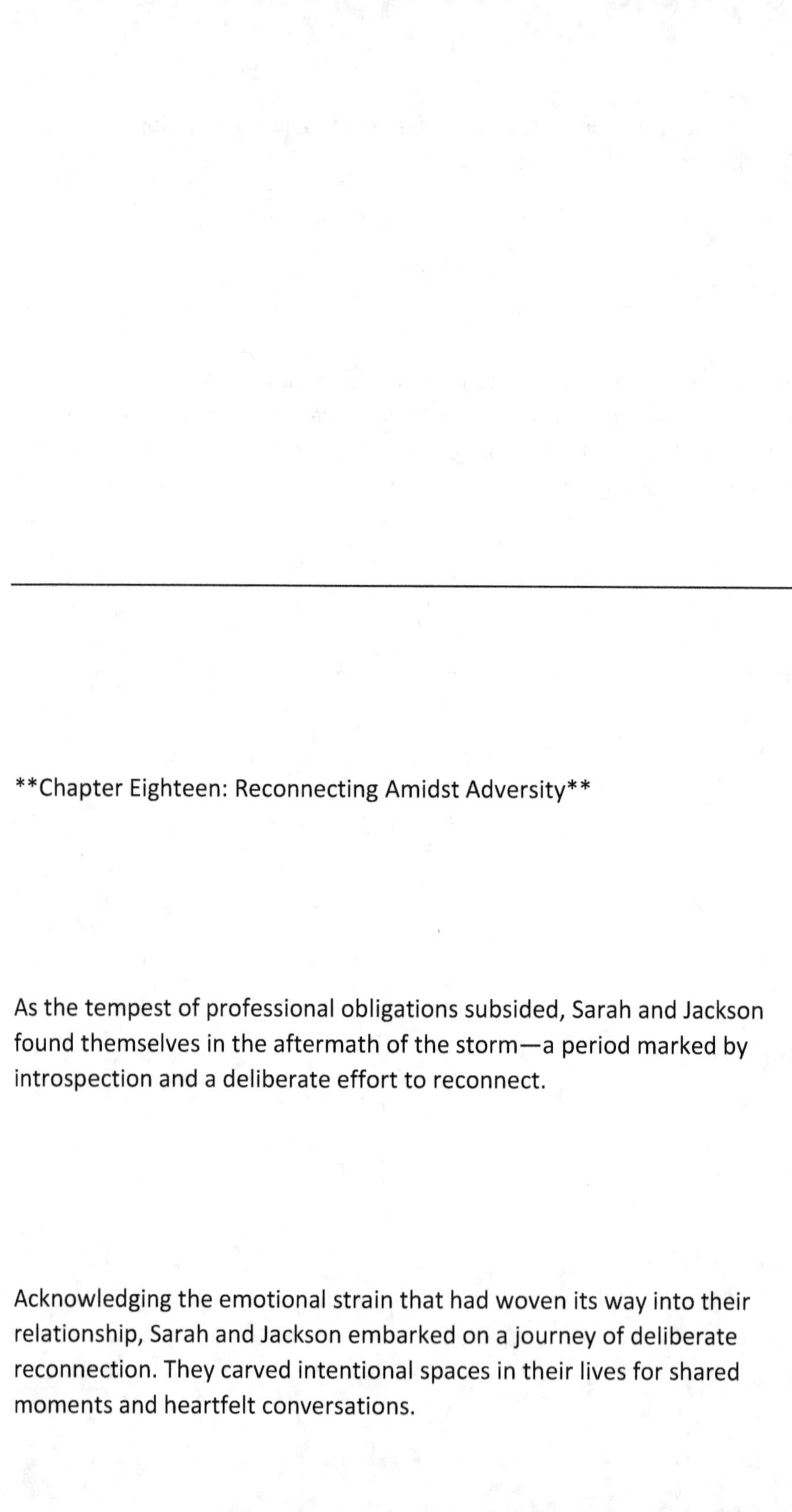

Chapter Eighteen: Reconnecting Amidst Adversity

As the tempest of professional obligations subsided, Sarah and Jackson found themselves in the aftermath of the storm—a period marked by introspection and a deliberate effort to reconnect.

Acknowledging the emotional strain that had woven its way into their relationship, Sarah and Jackson embarked on a journey of deliberate reconnection. They carved intentional spaces in their lives for shared moments and heartfelt conversations.

Through open communication and unwavering support, they navigated the remnants of the challenge, addressing the emotional distance that had momentarily clouded their connection. Their commitment to understanding and empathy became the cornerstone of their healing process.

In the sanctuary of shared vulnerability and mutual reassurance, Sarah and Jackson rediscovered the essence of their bond. Each conversation, each shared moment, served as a bridge that transcended the lingering shadows of the challenge they had faced.

Their intentional efforts to rebuild the bridges that connected their hearts breathed new life into their relationship. Through resilience and mutual understanding, they emerged from the challenge, their bond strengthened by the adversity they had bravely weathered together.

Chapter Nineteen: Rekindling Romance

Amidst the ebb and flow of life's demands, Sarah and Jackson found themselves intentional about rekindling the romantic essence of their relationship—an endeavor that breathed new life into their shared journey.

In the quietude of candlelit dinners and stolen moments, they immersed themselves in the artistry of romance. Jackson's thoughtful gestures and Sarah's tender affection became a symphony that echoed with the melody of their enduring love.

Their shared adventures took on hues of renewed passion—spontaneous getaways that mirrored the ardor of their blossoming romance, whispered confessions that reignited the sparks of affection, and shared passions that stoked the flames of their intimacy.

Through deliberate efforts and heartfelt gestures, Sarah and Jackson embraced the magic of romance, infusing their lives with the warmth of affection and the serenity of shared dreams. Their commitment to nurturing the romantic essence of their relationship breathed new vitality into their love story.

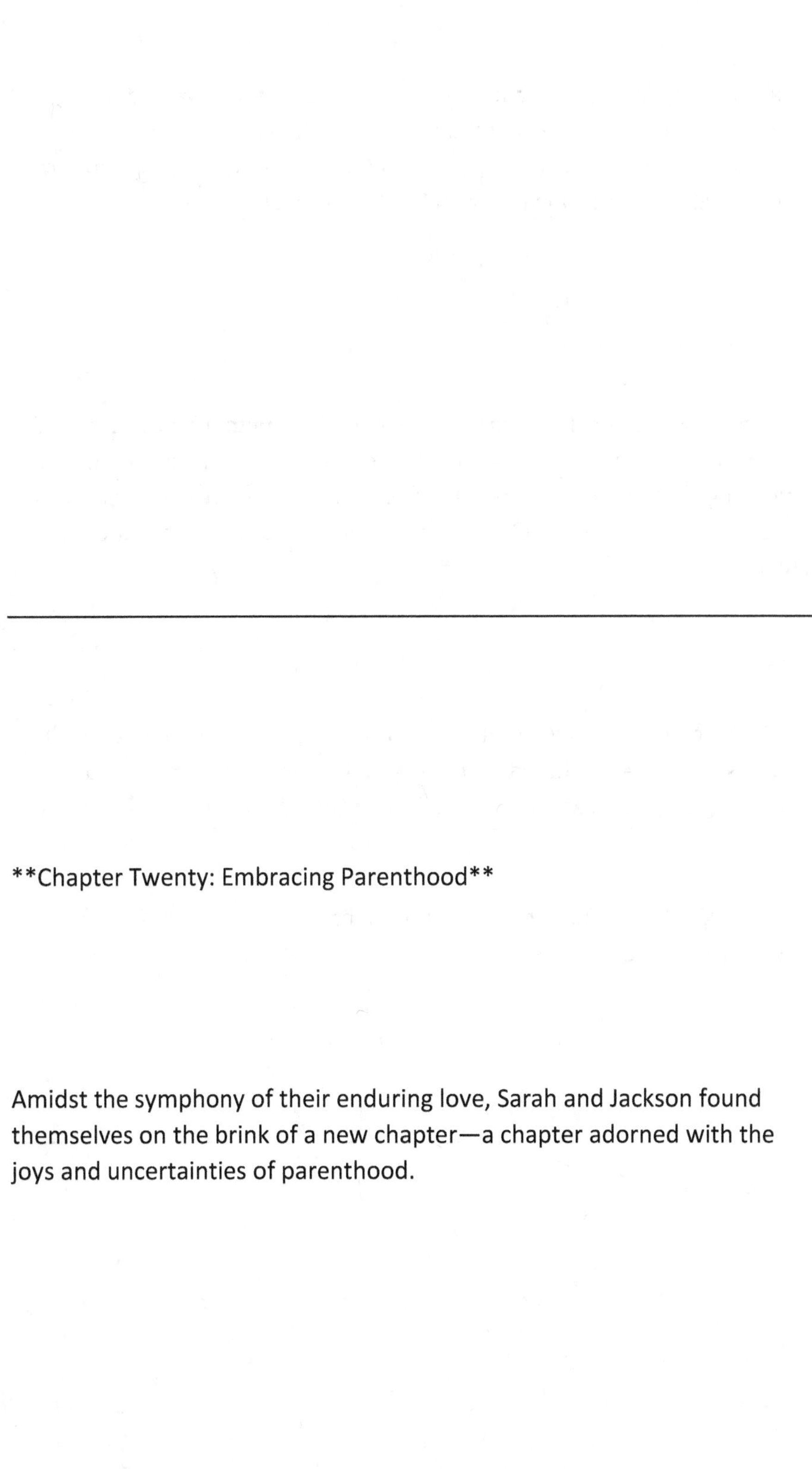

Chapter Twenty: Embracing Parenthood

Amidst the symphony of their enduring love, Sarah and Jackson found themselves on the brink of a new chapter—a chapter adorned with the joys and uncertainties of parenthood.

Their shared journey took a momentous turn as they embarked on the exhilarating path of expecting a child. Amidst the anticipation and excitement, Sarah's nurturing nature and Jackson's unwavering support became pillars upon which they embraced this new phase.

The anticipation of parenthood infused their lives with a renewed sense of purpose and unity. Together, they navigated the uncharted waters of preparing for the arrival of their little one—nurturing dreams, creating a haven, and envisioning a future embellished with the laughter of their child.

Their shared moments were imbued with tender gestures and heartfelt conversations, each interaction fueling their shared excitement and solidifying their unbreakable bond. Amidst the unknowns and

exhilaration, Sarah and Jackson found solace in their unwavering commitment to each other and their future family.

Chapter Twenty-One: Anticipation and Preparation

As the countdown to parenthood continued, Sarah and Jackson found themselves enveloped in the tender embrace of anticipation and preparation—a period marked by shared excitement and tender moments.

Their home transformed into a sanctuary of eager anticipation. Sarah's nurturing instinct blossomed as she meticulously prepared for their child's arrival, adorning their nest with love and care.

Together, they embarked on a journey of discovery, attending parenting classes, poring over parenting books, and reveling in the joyful chaos of assembling baby furniture. Each moment spent preparing for their child's arrival was an ode to their unwavering commitment to their growing family.

Conversations brimmed with excitement and dreams of the future—a future embellished with the pitter-patter of tiny feet and lullabies that would fill their home with the melody of parenthood.

Amidst the exhilaration, Sarah and Jackson's bond deepened, fortified by their shared dreams and anticipation. Their commitment to providing a nurturing environment for their child became a testament to the love and unity that defined their journey.

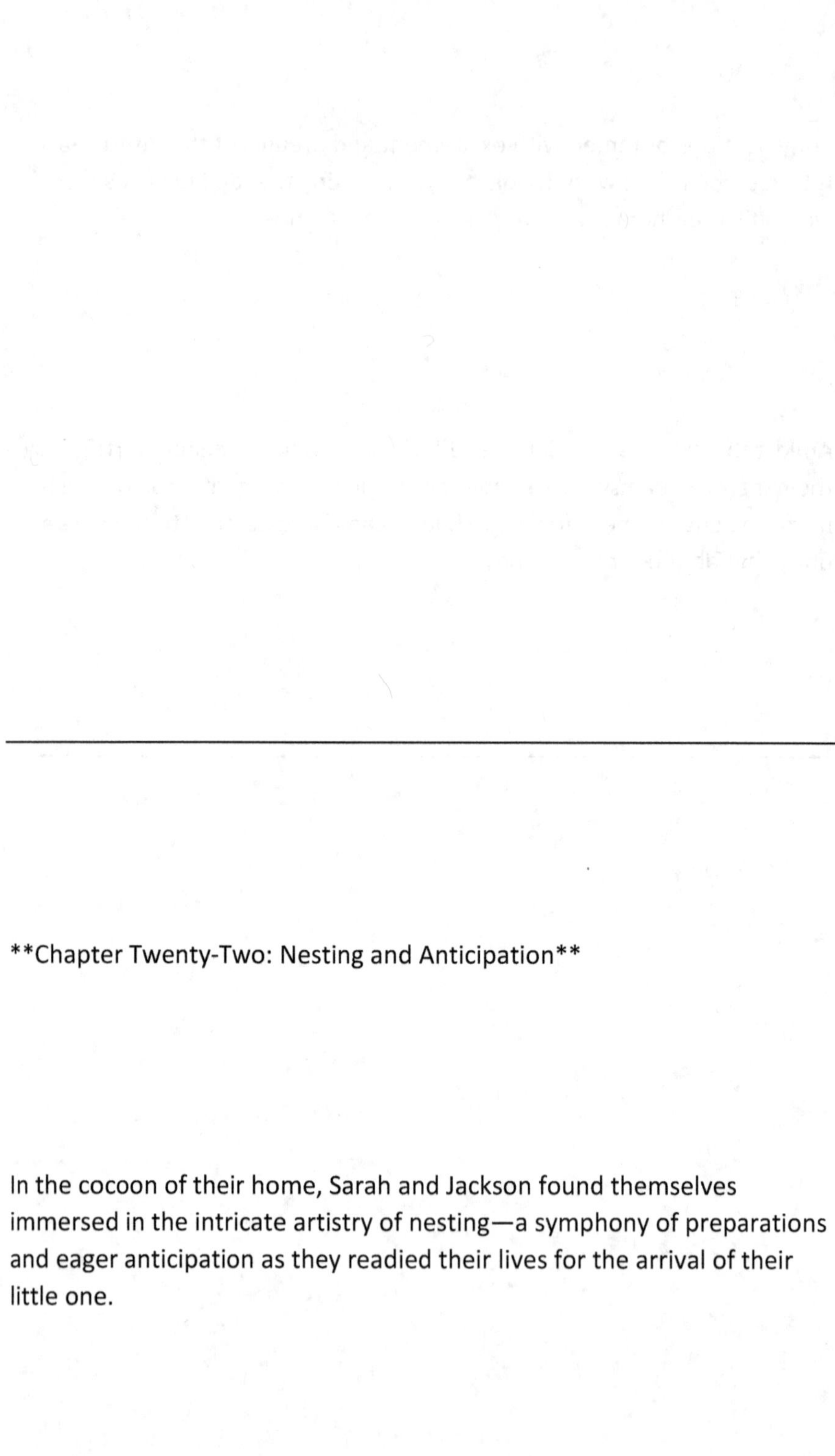

Chapter Twenty-Two: Nesting and Anticipation

In the cocoon of their home, Sarah and Jackson found themselves immersed in the intricate artistry of nesting—a symphony of preparations and eager anticipation as they readied their lives for the arrival of their little one.

The ambiance of their home transformed into a haven of meticulous planning and heartfelt gestures. Sarah's nurturing instinct flourished as she meticulously organized the nursery, adorning it with tender care and warmth.

Jackson, ever the doting partner, immersed himself in the preparations, channeling his unwavering dedication into ensuring that every corner of their home exuded comfort and security for their child.

Together, they embarked on a journey of anticipation—poring over parenting books, attending childbirth classes, and engaging in heartfelt conversations about their aspirations and dreams for their growing family.

Their home echoed with the melody of their shared excitement, each moment of preparation a testament to their unwavering commitment and boundless love for the little life soon to grace their world.

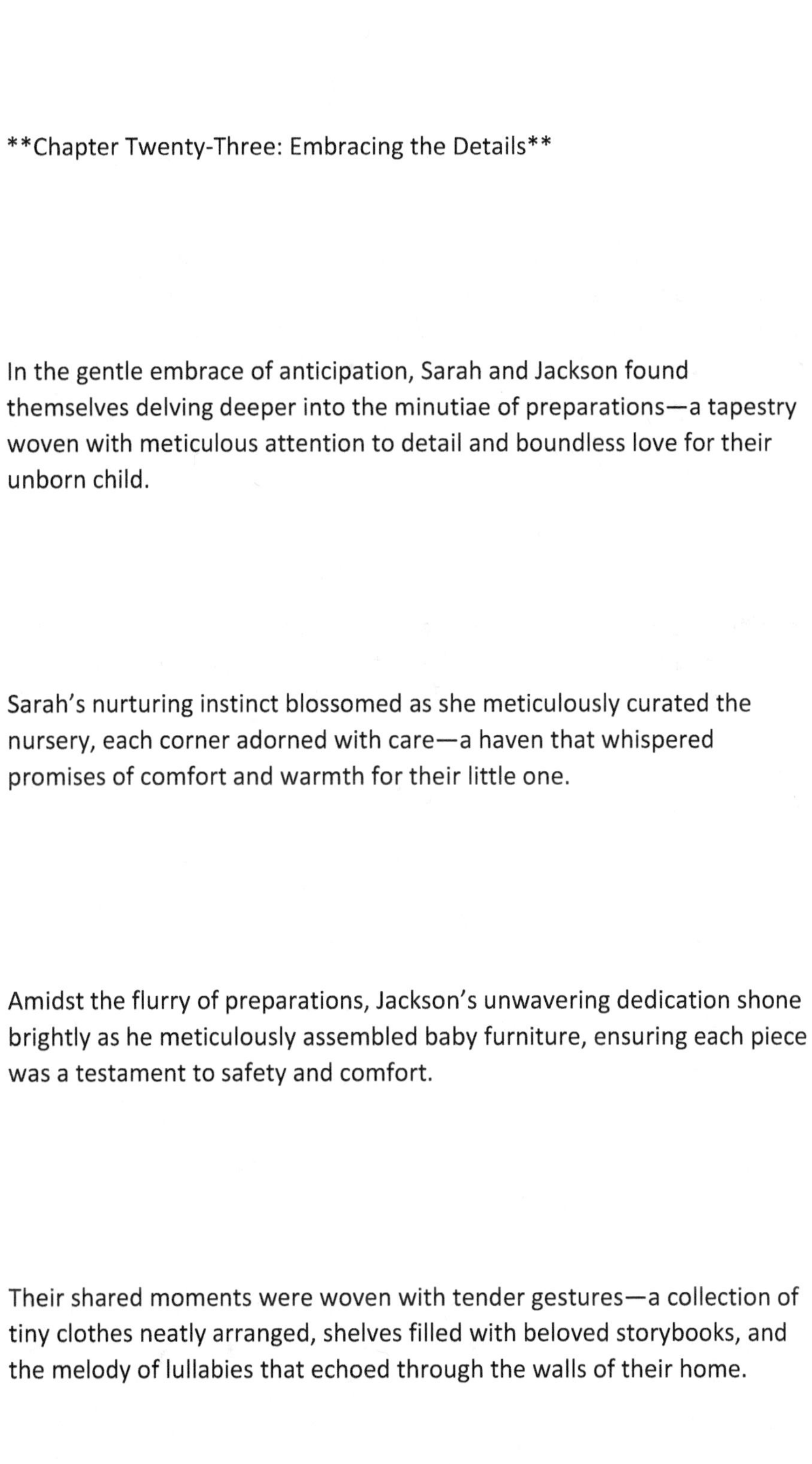

Chapter Twenty-Three: Embracing the Details

In the gentle embrace of anticipation, Sarah and Jackson found themselves delving deeper into the minutiae of preparations—a tapestry woven with meticulous attention to detail and boundless love for their unborn child.

Sarah's nurturing instinct blossomed as she meticulously curated the nursery, each corner adorned with care—a haven that whispered promises of comfort and warmth for their little one.

Amidst the flurry of preparations, Jackson's unwavering dedication shone brightly as he meticulously assembled baby furniture, ensuring each piece was a testament to safety and comfort.

Their shared moments were woven with tender gestures—a collection of tiny clothes neatly arranged, shelves filled with beloved storybooks, and the melody of lullabies that echoed through the walls of their home.

Conversations brimmed with excitement and earnest planning—discussions about parenting philosophies, shared aspirations, and the dreams they held for their child. Each decision, no matter how small, was imbued with their unified commitment to providing the best for their growing family.

Their home became a sanctuary of eager anticipation—a reflection of the love and dedication that filled their hearts as they meticulously prepared to welcome the newest member of their family.

Chapter Twenty-Four: Creating Memories

In the gentle embrace of nesting, Sarah and Jackson found themselves weaving intricate moments of preparation into cherished memories—a collage of thoughtful gestures and meticulous planning that painted their anticipation with vibrant hues.

Their home transformed into a sanctuary of love and preparation, every nook and cranny adorned with tender care. Sarah's nurturing touch resonated in every corner of the nursery, each item delicately chosen to create a cocoon of comfort for their soon-to-arrive bundle of joy.

Jackson, fueled by his unwavering commitment, meticulously crafted a haven, ensuring every detail in the nursery spoke volumes of security and warmth for their little one.

Together, they embarked on a journey of creating keepsakes—a collage of cherished moments captured in tiny onesies and soft blankets, shelves adorned with toys that promised laughter, and a crib that cradled dreams and aspirations for the future.

Their shared conversations were woven with joyful anticipation and earnest discussions about their parenting visions—philosophies steeped in love, respect, and the shared commitment to nurture and guide their child.

As they meticulously prepared their home, Sarah and Jackson forged bonds with each moment—a testament to the love and dedication that enveloped them as they eagerly awaited the arrival of their newest family member.

Chapter Twenty-Five: Cultivating Traditions

In the tender moments of preparation, Sarah and Jackson found themselves cultivating traditions—seeds of love and legacy planted amidst their meticulous arrangements, echoing promises of a nurturing home for their imminent arrival.

Their home metamorphosed into a canvas of cherished traditions and heartfelt rituals. Sarah's nurturing spirit resonated in every corner of the nursery, as she delicately curated a space that whispered promises of love and security for their little one.

Meanwhile, Jackson, driven by his unwavering devotion, crafted a sanctuary—a haven meticulously designed to envelop their child in comfort and warmth.

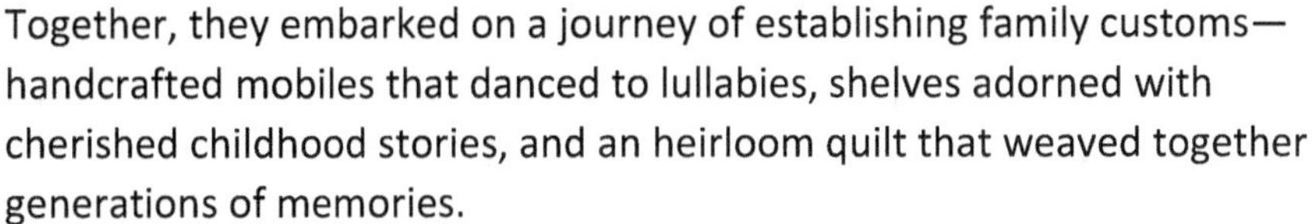

Together, they embarked on a journey of establishing family customs—handcrafted mobiles that danced to lullabies, shelves adorned with cherished childhood stories, and an heirloom quilt that weaved together generations of memories.

Their shared moments became a tapestry woven with laughter and heartfelt conversations, each decision made with an unwavering commitment to fostering an environment filled with love, laughter, and cherished family traditions.

As they meticulously prepared their home, Sarah and Jackson forged bonds with each cherished tradition—a testament to the love and dedication that enveloped them as they eagerly anticipated the arrival of their newest family member.

Chapter Twenty-Six: Crafting Dreams

Amidst the anticipation of new beginnings, Sarah and Jackson found themselves crafting dreams—each gesture, every meticulous arrangement, a testament to their unwavering commitment to creating a haven for their growing family.

Their home transformed into a sanctuary of love and dreams. Sarah's nurturing touch graced every corner of the nursery, weaving a tapestry of comfort and warmth for their little one.

Meanwhile, Jackson's meticulous efforts ensured that every detail, from the softest blankets to the gentlest nightlights, painted a picture of security and serenity for their child.

Together, they embarked on a journey of envisioning shared aspirations—a collection of bedtime stories waiting to be told, a tiny pair of footprints leaving imprints on the heart, and a world of possibilities awaiting their little one.

Their shared moments became a mosaic of anticipation and tender affection, every decision crafted with an unwavering commitment to shaping a future filled with love, support, and boundless dreams.

As they meticulously prepared their home, Sarah and Jackson carved the foundation for their dreams—a testament to the love and dedication that enveloped them as they eagerly awaited the arrival of their newest family member.

Chapter Twenty-Seven: Envisioning Parenthood

In the crescendo of their anticipation, Sarah and Jackson found themselves envisioning the remarkable journey of parenthood—a tapestry woven with intricacy and adorned with the promises of unconditional love and endless possibilities.

Their home became a sanctuary of tender dreams and heartwarming aspirations. Sarah's nurturing touch graced every detail of the nursery, meticulously creating an atmosphere cocooned in love and tenderness for their little one.

Concurrently, Jackson's unwavering commitment was reflected in every corner, where his meticulous efforts crafted a haven brimming with safety and warmth, ready to welcome their child into the world.

Together, they embarked on a profound journey of envisioning the moments to come—a future adorned with lullabies echoing in the air, tiny footsteps exploring the uncharted, and heartfelt whispers of guidance and encouragement.

Their shared moments became an exquisite panorama of joyful anticipation, every decision made with unwavering dedication to ushering in a world of boundless love and endless opportunities for their beloved child.

As they meticulously prepared their home, Sarah and Jackson set the stage for a lifetime of love and wonder—a testament to the deep affection and devoted preparations that enveloped them as they eagerly anticipated the arrival of their newest family member.

Chapter Twenty-Eight: Embracing New Beginnings

As the much-awaited moment drew near, Sarah and Jackson found themselves on the brink of a new chapter—a chapter illuminated by the radiant arrival of their precious child, heralding the dawn of parenthood.

Their home, a sanctuary meticulously prepared with tender care, resonated with the anticipation of new beginnings. Sarah's nurturing instinct permeated every detail, creating a haven exuding warmth and comfort for their little one.

Meanwhile, Jackson's steadfast dedication ensured that every corner radiated security and love, ready to cradle their child in an embrace of safety and warmth.

Together, they stood at the threshold of a profound transformation—anticipating the transformative joy that awaited them as they embraced the journey of nurturing, guiding, and cherishing their newborn.

Their shared moments brimmed with overwhelming joy and heartfelt eagerness, every breath a testament to their profound love and unwavering commitment to embracing the beautiful journey of parenthood.

As they eagerly awaited the arrival of their child, Sarah and Jackson stood united in anticipation, ready to embark on the remarkable journey of raising and nurturing their little one—a testament to the depth of their love and the radiant possibilities that awaited them.

Chapter Twenty-Nine: The Miracle of New Life

Amidst the serenity of their home, Sarah and Jackson stood on the precipice of a transformative chapter—the arrival of their newborn—a moment enveloped in the sheer wonder and miracle of new life.

The ambiance of their home radiated with palpable anticipation. Every corner, meticulously arranged and tenderly prepared, whispered promises of comfort and security for their awaited little one.

Sarah, brimming with a mother's love, found solace in the nursery she had curated with meticulous care—a haven that echoed her nurturing spirit, ready to embrace the newborn in a cocoon of warmth.

Meanwhile, Jackson's steadfast dedication ensured that every detail, from the gentlest cribs to the softest blankets, exuded an aura of safety and love, awaiting the arrival of their child.

Together, they embraced the tender expectancy of imminent parenthood—a phase adorned with shared hopes, joyful expectations, and the humbling awe of witnessing the miracle of new life.

Their shared moments resonated with a profound sense of unity, each heartbeat echoing the anticipation of the life-altering journey that awaited them—the breathtaking voyage of nurturing, cherishing, and guiding their beloved child.

As they stood united in the anticipation of their newborn's arrival, Sarah and Jackson brimmed with boundless love and unspoken promises of devotion—a testament to the awe-inspiring beauty of embarking on the sacred journey of parenthood.

Chapter Thirty: Embracing the First Moments

In the hushed tranquility of their home, Sarah and Jackson found themselves immersed in the ethereal moments following the arrival of their newborn—a chapter adorned with tender discoveries and the irreplaceable essence of new beginnings.

Their home, once a sanctuary of eager anticipation, now resonated with the melody of gentle lullabies and the soothing whispers of parental affection. Every corner, meticulously arranged, cocooned their newborn in a cradle of comfort and security.

Sarah, radiant with the glow of motherhood, reveled in the sacred bond she nurtured with their newborn—a testament to her unconditional love and unwavering dedication.

Meanwhile, Jackson's tender devotion painted every moment with paternal warmth—a beacon of support and affection that embraced their child in a haven of safety and love.

Together, they embarked on the enchanting voyage of discovery—a symphony of firsts, from the delicate touch of tiny fingers to the heartwarming lullabies that filled the air with serenity.

Their shared moments became a tapestry woven with love and awe, each breath a celebration of the cherished milestones and the overwhelming joy that graced their newfound journey of parenthood.

As they basked in the glow of these precious moments, Sarah and Jackson stood united in the magnificence of witnessing life's miracles—a testament to the boundless love and unspoken promises that adorned their path as they embraced the captivating journey of parenthood.

Chapter Thirty-One: Nurturing Bonds

Amidst the tender embrace of parenthood, Sarah and Jackson found themselves immersed in the artistry of nurturing—the delicate dance of bonding, fostering a connection that transcended time and words.

Their home, now a cradle of love and discovery, echoed with the harmonious melody of parental devotion. Every moment, every tender caress, was a testament to the unspoken promises of care and unconditional love.

Sarah, adorned with the grace of motherhood, found solace in the symphony of their shared moments—a testament to her unwavering dedication to nurturing and cherishing their child.

Simultaneously, Jackson's paternal warmth enveloped their home—a steady presence filled with tenderness and guidance, fostering an environment steeped in security and affection.

Together, they embarked on the enchanting voyage of parenthood—a tapestry woven with tender lullabies, whispered promises of protection, and a myriad of shared discoveries.

Their shared moments became the threads of an unbreakable bond, each smile, each embrace, a testament to the profound connection they forged as they embraced the captivating journey of nurturing their child.

As they reveled in the tender beauty of parenthood, Sarah and Jackson stood united in their commitment—a testament to the boundless love and unwavering dedication that adorned their path as they cherished the breathtaking journey of nurturing their growing family.

Chapter Thirty-Two: Midnight Serenade

Amidst the quietude of their home, Sarah and Jackson found themselves entwined in the enchanting symphony of midnight serenades—a chapter painted with tender moments and shared rituals that defined their journey as new parents.

Their home, once cloaked in hushed whispers, now reverberated with the soft melodies of lullabies and the gentle coos of their little one. Each night became a tableau of warmth and affection, a sacred ritual of nurturing and soothing their child.

Sarah, illuminated by the glow of motherhood, cradled their baby in loving arms, weaving a cocoon of comfort and security with each tender embrace.

Meanwhile, Jackson, unwavering in his paternal devotion, stood by her side—a pillar of support and reassurance, lending his gentle touch to the soothing rhythm of their nighttime ritual.

Together, they danced in the silent cadence of parenthood—a choreography of shared moments, whispered assurances, and a profound understanding that bloomed amidst the tranquil hours of the night.

Their shared serenades became an ode to the unspoken bond they nurtured, each whispered lullaby a testament to the depth of their love and dedication as they embraced the tender yet powerful role of guiding and comforting their precious child through the quiet hours.

As they waltzed through the nocturnal symphony, Sarah and Jackson found solace in their unity—a testament to the timeless love and devotion that adorned their path as they embraced the ethereal journey of parenthood.

Chapter Thirty-Three: The Dance of Patience

Amidst the gentle rhythm of their home, Sarah and Jackson found themselves engaged in the intricate dance of patience—a testament to their unwavering commitment and resilience as they navigated the challenges of parenthood.

Their home, a sanctuary of love and learning, echoed with the symphony of a baby's cries and the delicate footsteps of adjustment. Each moment was a canvas of growth, patience, and the artistry of understanding their little one's needs.

Sarah, adorned with the grace of maternal instinct, embraced the trials with unwavering tenderness and patience—a beacon of comfort and reassurance for their child.

Meanwhile, Jackson, steadfast in his paternal role, stood by her side—a pillar of support and understanding, lending his unwavering patience to the delicate choreography of parenthood.

Together, they waltzed through the challenges, embracing the teachable moments and nurturing an environment steeped in love, patience, and understanding.

Their shared experiences became a testimony to the strength of their unity—a harmony of understanding and resilience that emerged amidst the trials and joys of guiding and nurturing their growing family.

As they danced through the intricacies of patience, Sarah and Jackson found solace in their partnership—a testament to their enduring love and dedication as they embraced the humbling yet empowering journey of parenthood.

Chapter Twenty-Four: Creating Memories

In the gentle embrace of nesting, Sarah and Jackson found themselves weaving intricate moments of preparation into cherished memories—a collage of thoughtful gestures and meticulous planning that painted their anticipation with vibrant hues.

Their home transformed into a sanctuary of love and preparation, every nook and cranny adorned with tender care. Sarah's nurturing touch resonated in every corner of the nursery, each item delicately chosen to create a cocoon of comfort for their soon-to-arrive bundle of joy.

Jackson, fueled by his unwavering commitment, meticulously crafted a haven, ensuring every detail in the nursery spoke volumes of security and warmth for their little one.

Together, they embarked on a journey of creating keepsakes—a collage of cherished moments captured in tiny onesies and soft blankets, shelves adorned with toys that promised laughter, and a crib that cradled dreams and aspirations for the future.

Their shared conversations were woven with joyful anticipation and earnest discussions about their parenting visions—philosophies steeped in love, respect, and the shared commitment to nurture and guide their child.

As they meticulously prepared their home, Sarah and Jackson forged bonds with each moment—a testament to the love and dedication that enveloped them as they eagerly awaited the arrival of their newest family member.

Chapter Twenty-Five: Cultivating Traditions

In the tender moments of preparation, Sarah and Jackson found themselves cultivating traditions—seeds of love and legacy planted amidst their meticulous arrangements, echoing promises of a nurturing home for their imminent arrival.

Their home metamorphosed into a canvas of cherished traditions and heartfelt rituals. Sarah's nurturing spirit resonated in every corner of the nursery, as she delicately curated a space that whispered promises of love and security for their little one.

Meanwhile, Jackson, driven by his unwavering devotion, crafted a sanctuary—a haven meticulously designed to envelop their child in comfort and warmth.

Together, they embarked on a journey of establishing family customs—handcrafted mobiles that danced to lullabies, shelves adorned with cherished childhood stories, and an heirloom quilt that weaved together generations of memories.

Their shared moments became a tapestry woven with laughter and heartfelt conversations, each decision made with an unwavering commitment to fostering an environment filled with love, laughter, and cherished family traditions.

As they meticulously prepared their home, Sarah and Jackson forged bonds with each cherished tradition—a testament to the love and dedication that enveloped them as they eagerly anticipated the arrival of their newest family member.

Chapter Twenty-Six: Crafting Dreams

Amidst the anticipation of new beginnings, Sarah and Jackson found themselves crafting dreams—each gesture, every meticulous arrangement, a testament to their unwavering commitment to creating a haven for their growing family.

Their home transformed into a sanctuary of love and dreams. Sarah's nurturing touch graced every corner of the nursery, weaving a tapestry of comfort and warmth for their little one.

Meanwhile, Jackson's meticulous efforts ensured that every detail, from the softest blankets to the gentlest nightlights, painted a picture of security and serenity for their child.

Together, they embarked on a journey of envisioning shared aspirations—a collection of bedtime stories waiting to be told, a tiny pair of footprints

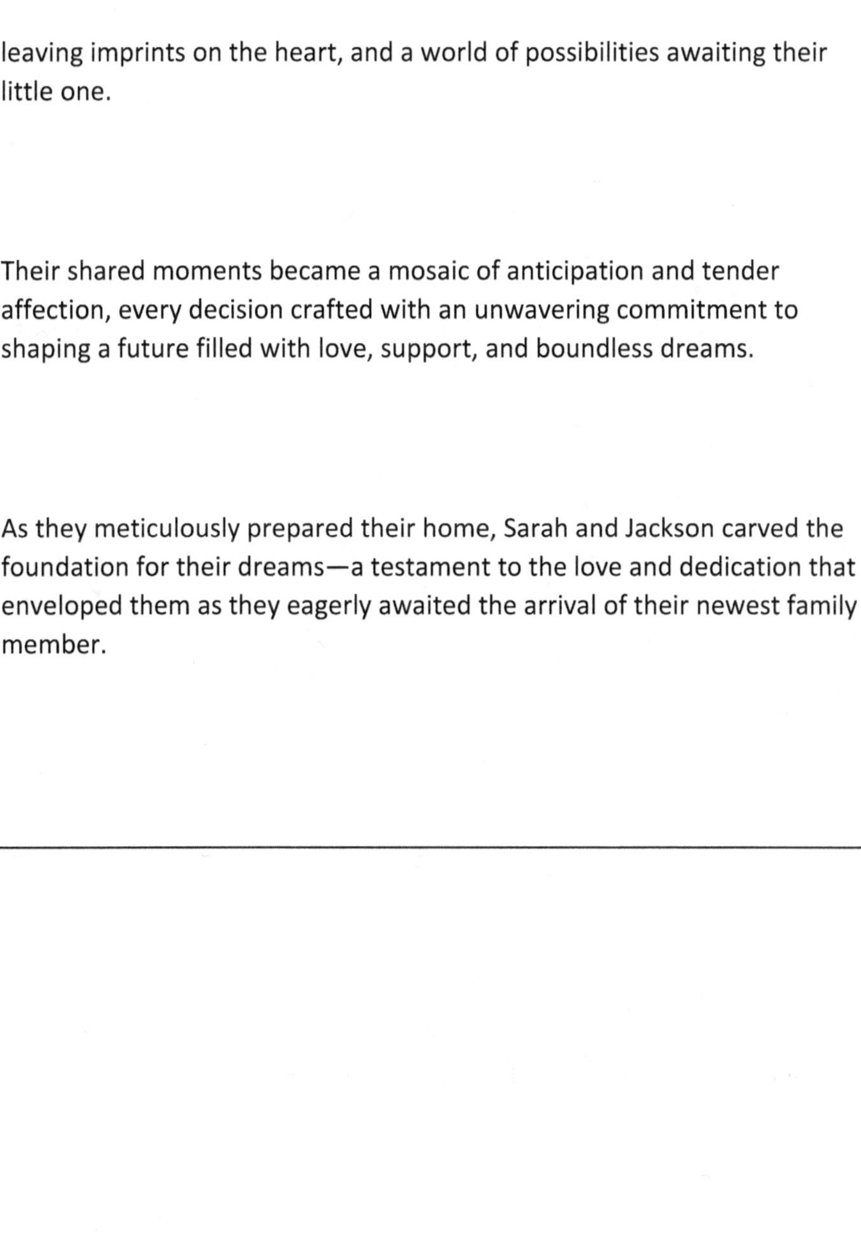

leaving imprints on the heart, and a world of possibilities awaiting their little one.

Their shared moments became a mosaic of anticipation and tender affection, every decision crafted with an unwavering commitment to shaping a future filled with love, support, and boundless dreams.

As they meticulously prepared their home, Sarah and Jackson carved the foundation for their dreams—a testament to the love and dedication that enveloped them as they eagerly awaited the arrival of their newest family member.

Chapter Twenty-Seven: Envisioning Parenthood

In the crescendo of their anticipation, Sarah and Jackson found themselves envisioning the remarkable journey of parenthood—a tapestry woven with intricacy and adorned with the promises of unconditional love and endless possibilities.

Their home became a sanctuary of tender dreams and heartwarming aspirations. Sarah's nurturing touch graced every detail of the nursery, meticulously creating an atmosphere cocooned in love and tenderness for their little one.

Concurrently, Jackson's unwavering commitment was reflected in every corner, where his meticulous efforts crafted a haven brimming with safety and warmth, ready to welcome their child into the world.

Together, they embarked on a profound journey of envisioning the moments to come—a future adorned with lullabies echoing in the air, tiny footsteps exploring the uncharted, and heartfelt whispers of guidance and encouragement.

Their shared moments became an exquisite panorama of joyful anticipation, every decision made with unwavering dedication to ushering in a world of boundless love and endless opportunities for their beloved child.

As they meticulously prepared their home, Sarah and Jackson set the stage for a lifetime of love and wonder—a testament to the deep affection and devoted preparations that enveloped them as they eagerly anticipated the arrival of their newest family member.

Chapter Twenty-Eight: Embracing New Beginnings

As the much-awaited moment drew near, Sarah and Jackson found themselves on the brink of a new chapter—a chapter illuminated by the radiant arrival of their precious child, heralding the dawn of parenthood.

Their home, a sanctuary meticulously prepared with tender care, resonated with the anticipation of new beginnings. Sarah's nurturing instinct permeated every detail, creating a haven exuding warmth and comfort for their little one.

Meanwhile, Jackson's steadfast dedication ensured that every corner radiated security and love, ready to cradle their child in an embrace of safety and warmth.

Together, they stood at the threshold of a profound transformation—anticipating the transformative joy that awaited them as they embraced the journey of nurturing, guiding, and cherishing their newborn.

Their shared moments brimmed with overwhelming joy and heartfelt eagerness, every breath a testament to their profound love and unwavering commitment to embracing the beautiful journey of parenthood.

As they eagerly awaited the arrival of their child, Sarah and Jackson stood united in anticipation, ready to embark on the remarkable journey of raising and nurturing their little one—a testament to the depth of their love and the radiant possibilities that awaited them.

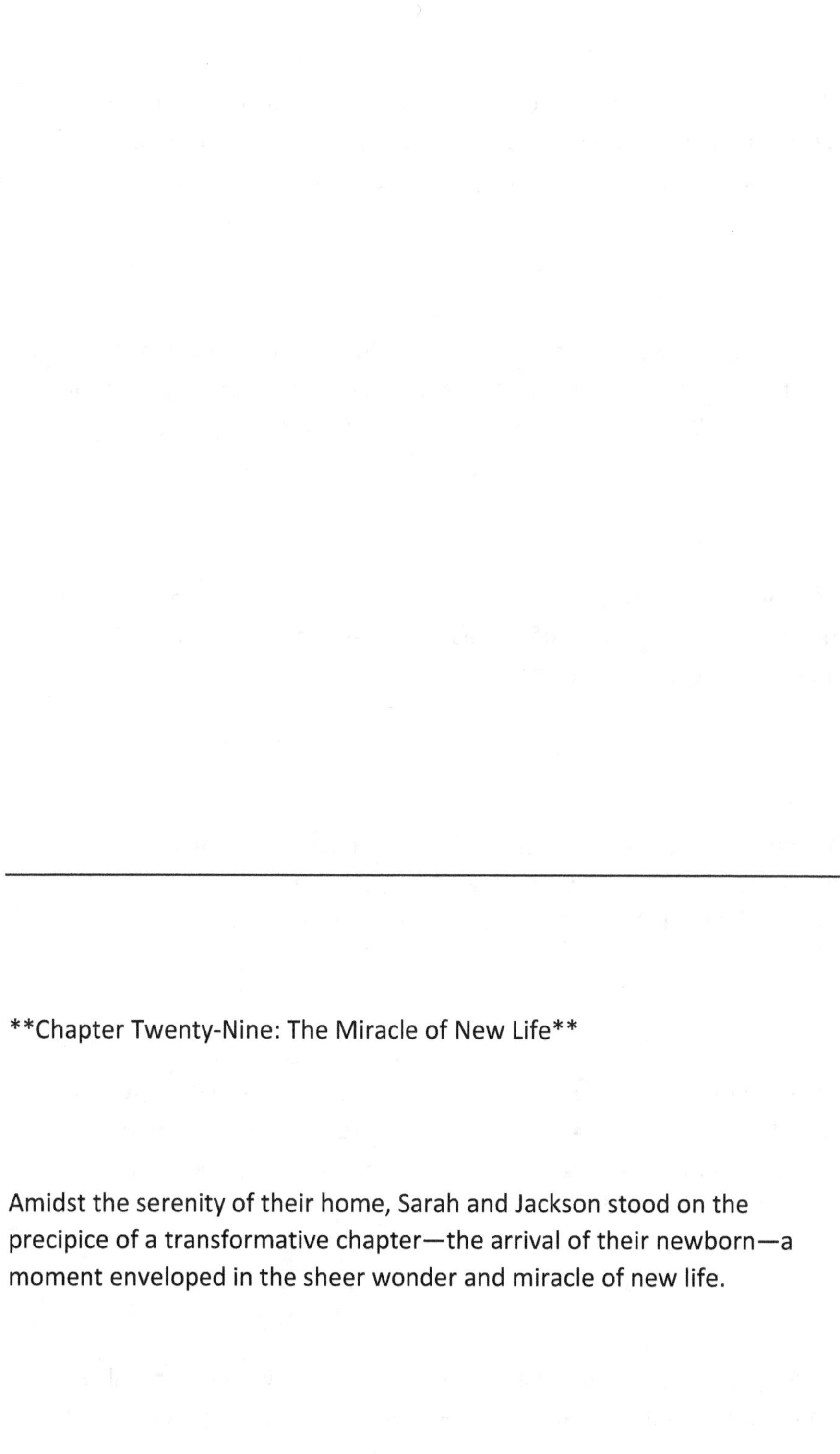

Chapter Twenty-Nine: The Miracle of New Life

Amidst the serenity of their home, Sarah and Jackson stood on the precipice of a transformative chapter—the arrival of their newborn—a moment enveloped in the sheer wonder and miracle of new life.

The ambiance of their home radiated with palpable anticipation. Every corner, meticulously arranged and tenderly prepared, whispered promises of comfort and security for their awaited little one.

Sarah, brimming with a mother's love, found solace in the nursery she had curated with meticulous care—a haven that echoed her nurturing spirit, ready to embrace the newborn in a cocoon of warmth.

Meanwhile, Jackson's steadfast dedication ensured that every detail, from the gentlest cribs to the softest blankets, exuded an aura of safety and love, awaiting the arrival of their child.

Together, they embraced the tender expectancy of imminent parenthood—a phase adorned with shared hopes, joyful expectations, and the humbling awe of witnessing the miracle of new life.

Their shared moments resonated with a profound sense of unity, each heartbeat echoing the anticipation of the life-altering journey that awaited them—the breathtaking voyage of nurturing, cherishing, and guiding their beloved child.

As they stood united in the anticipation of their newborn's arrival, Sarah and Jackson brimmed with boundless love and unspoken promises of devotion—a testament to the awe-inspiring beauty of embarking on the sacred journey of parenthood.

Chapter Thirty: Embracing the First Moments

In the hushed tranquility of their home, Sarah and Jackson found themselves immersed in the ethereal moments following the arrival of their newborn—a chapter adorned with tender discoveries and the irreplaceable essence of new beginnings.

Their home, once a sanctuary of eager anticipation, now resonated with the melody of gentle lullabies and the soothing whispers of parental affection. Every corner, meticulously arranged, cocooned their newborn in a cradle of comfort and security.

Sarah, radiant with the glow of motherhood, reveled in the sacred bond she nurtured with their newborn—a testament to her unconditional love and unwavering dedication.

Meanwhile, Jackson's tender devotion painted every moment with paternal warmth—a beacon of support and affection that embraced their child in a haven of safety and love.

Together, they embarked on the enchanting voyage of discovery—a symphony of firsts, from the delicate touch of tiny fingers to the heartwarming lullabies that filled the air with serenity.

Their shared moments became a tapestry woven with love and awe, each breath a celebration of the cherished milestones and the overwhelming joy that graced their newfound journey of parenthood.

As they basked in the glow of these precious moments, Sarah and Jackson stood united in the magnificence of witnessing life's miracles—a testament to the boundless love and unspoken promises that adorned their path as they embraced the captivating journey of parenthood.

Chapter Thirty-One: Nurturing Bonds

Amidst the tender embrace of parenthood, Sarah and Jackson found themselves immersed in the artistry of nurturing—the delicate dance of bonding, fostering a connection that transcended time and words.

Their home, now a cradle of love and discovery, echoed with the harmonious melody of parental devotion. Every moment, every tender caress, was a testament to the unspoken promises of care and unconditional love.

Sarah, adorned with the grace of motherhood, found solace in the symphony of their shared moments—a testament to her unwavering dedication to nurturing and cherishing their child.

Simultaneously, Jackson's paternal warmth enveloped their home—a steady presence filled with tenderness and guidance, fostering an environment steeped in security and affection.

Together, they embarked on the enchanting voyage of parenthood—a tapestry woven with tender lullabies, whispered promises of protection, and a myriad of shared discoveries.

Their shared moments became the threads of an unbreakable bond, each smile, each embrace, a testament to the profound connection they forged as they embraced the captivating journey of nurturing their child.

As they reveled in the tender beauty of parenthood, Sarah and Jackson stood united in their commitment—a testament to the boundless love and unwavering dedication that adorned their path as they cherished the breathtaking journey of nurturing their growing family.

Chapter Thirty-Two: Midnight Serenade

Amidst the quietude of their home, Sarah and Jackson found themselves entwined in the enchanting symphony of midnight serenades—a chapter painted with tender moments and shared rituals that defined their journey as new parents.

Their home, once cloaked in hushed whispers, now reverberated with the soft melodies of lullabies and the gentle coos of their little one. Each night became a tableau of warmth and affection, a sacred ritual of nurturing and soothing their child.

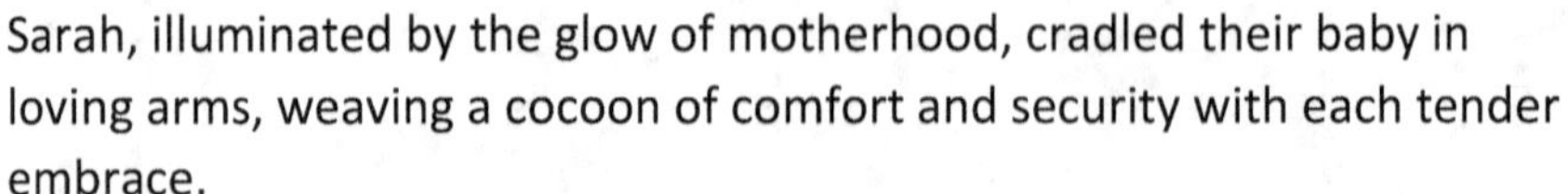

Sarah, illuminated by the glow of motherhood, cradled their baby in loving arms, weaving a cocoon of comfort and security with each tender embrace.

Meanwhile, Jackson, unwavering in his paternal devotion, stood by her side—a pillar of support and reassurance, lending his gentle touch to the soothing rhythm of their nighttime ritual.

Together, they danced in the silent cadence of parenthood—a choreography of shared moments, whispered assurances, and a profound understanding that bloomed amidst the tranquil hours of the night.

Their shared serenades became an ode to the unspoken bond they nurtured, each whispered lullaby a testament to the depth of their love and dedication as they embraced the tender yet powerful role of guiding and comforting their precious child through the quiet hours.

As they waltzed through the nocturnal symphony, Sarah and Jackson found solace in their unity—a testament to the timeless love and devotion that adorned their path as they embraced the ethereal journey of parenthood.

____

Chapter Thirty-Three: The Dance of Patience

Amidst the gentle rhythm of their home, Sarah and Jackson found themselves engaged in the intricate dance of patience—a testament to their unwavering commitment and resilience as they navigated the challenges of parenthood.

Their home, a sanctuary of love and learning, echoed with the symphony of a baby's cries and the delicate footsteps of adjustment. Each moment was a canvas of growth, patience, and the artistry of understanding their little one's needs.

Sarah, adorned with the grace of maternal instinct, embraced the trials with unwavering tenderness and patience—a beacon of comfort and reassurance for their child.

Meanwhile, Jackson, steadfast in his paternal role, stood by her side—a pillar of support and understanding, lending his unwavering patience to the delicate choreography of parenthood.

Together, they waltzed through the challenges, embracing the teachable moments and nurturing an environment steeped in love, patience, and understanding.

Their shared experiences became a testimony to the strength of their unity—a harmony of understanding and resilience that emerged amidst the trials and joys of guiding and nurturing their growing family.

As they danced through the intricacies of patience, Sarah and Jackson found solace in their partnership—a testament to their enduring love and dedication as they embraced the humbling yet empowering journey of parenthood.

Chapter Thirty-Four: The Language of Firsts

Amidst the tender embrace of their home, Sarah and Jackson found themselves fluent in the language of firsts—a captivating symphony of milestones and cherished moments that adorned their journey as parents.

Their home, a sanctuary of discovery, echoed with the exuberance of their little one's laughter and the exhilarating crescendo of milestones achieved. Each moment was a testament to growth, wonder, and the joy of witnessing their child's firsts.

Sarah, adorned with the wonder of motherhood, savored every moment—a witness to the first smiles, the tentative steps, and the babbled words that painted the canvas of their child's growth.

Meanwhile, Jackson, anchored in the pride of fatherhood, embraced each milestone—a steadfast supporter, celebrating the triumphs and comforting through the challenges that marked their child's journey.

Together, they reveled in the enchanting journey of firsts—a tapestry woven with joyous celebrations, heartfelt applause, and the immeasurable pride that came with nurturing and guiding their little one through these monumental moments.

Their shared experiences became an anthem to the beauty of parenthood—a testament to the awe-inspiring privilege of witnessing and nurturing the tender milestones that shaped their growing family.

As they conversed in the language of firsts, Sarah and Jackson found solace in their shared delight—a testament to their boundless love and profound dedication as they reveled in the enchanting journey of parenthood.

Chapter Thirty-Five: Finding Balance

Amidst the whirlwind of their home, Sarah and Jackson found themselves in pursuit of balance—a delicate dance of juggling responsibilities while savoring the moments that define their journey as parents.

Their home, once a sanctuary of quietude, now resonated with the joyful chaos of family life. Every moment was a blend of nurturing, learning, and the art of finding equilibrium in the midst of parenthood.

Sarah, adorned with the grace of multitasking, embraced the challenges with determination—a testament to her resilience in balancing the roles of caregiver, partner, and nurturer.

Meanwhile, Jackson, steadfast in his commitment, maneuvered through the demands—a reliable presence, sharing the responsibilities and joys, ensuring a harmonious environment for their family.

Together, they navigated the complexities—a symphony of compromise, shared duties, and cherished moments, striving to strike a balance between tending to their child's needs and nurturing their relationship.

Their shared experiences became a testament to their unity—a fusion of understanding and support that fortified their bond as they embraced the rewarding yet demanding journey of parenthood.

As they sought equilibrium amidst the bustling rhythm of family life, Sarah and Jackson found solace in their unity—a testament to their enduring love and unwavering dedication as they navigated the beautiful complexities of parenthood.

Chapter Thirty-Six: Building Dreams Together

In the heart of their home, Sarah and Jackson found themselves united in the pursuit of shared achievements—a testament to their resilience, unity, and unwavering commitment as they journeyed through the tapestry of parenthood.

Their home, a haven of dreams and aspirations, echoed with the echoes of shared accomplishments and the triumphant steps taken together. Each milestone they reached was a testament to their mutual support and shared determination.

Sarah, adorned with the resilience of motherhood, led with unwavering dedication—a beacon of strength and inspiration, laying the foundation for their child's future with steadfast resolve.

Meanwhile, Jackson, anchored in his paternal role, stood shoulder to shoulder—a steadfast partner, sharing the triumphs and weathering the storms, nurturing their child's growth and supporting Sarah through every step.

Together, they forged a path—a symphony of shared dreams, a collection of achievements, and a testament to their unbreakable bond as they worked hand in hand, nurturing their family and fostering an environment brimming with love and opportunity.

Their shared accomplishments became a testament to their unity—a testament to the enduring love, dedication, and resilience that marked their journey as they nurtured their growing family and built their dreams together.

Chapter Thirty-Seven: Embracing Victories

Amidst the bustling rhythm of their home, Sarah and Jackson found themselves adorned with the laurels of shared victories—a testament to their resilience, unity, and the remarkable milestones they achieved together in their parenthood journey.

Their home, once a canvas of dreams, resonated with the echoes of triumphs and shared accomplishments. Each milestone reached was a testament to their dedication, perseverance, and unwavering commitment to their growing family.

Sarah, adorned with the strength of motherhood, led with unwavering resolve—a guiding light and a nurturer of dreams, fostering an environment steeped in love and opportunity for their child.

Meanwhile, Jackson, anchored in his paternal role, stood as an unwavering ally—a partner in every victory, supporting and celebrating alongside Sarah, ensuring their child had the best foundation for growth and success.

Together, they celebrated achievements—a symphony of shared joys, a chorus of resilience, and a testament to their unbreakable bond as they nurtured their family and witnessed the beautiful fruits of their labor.

Their shared victories became a testament to their unity—a celebration of enduring love, dedication, and the resilience that marked their journey as they fostered a nurturing environment and embraced the milestones of their growing family.

Chapter Thirty-Eight: Cultivating Gratitude

In the tranquility of their home, Sarah and Jackson found themselves immersed in the practice of gratitude—a cornerstone of their parenthood journey, shaping their perspectives and fostering a culture of appreciation.

Their home, a sanctuary of mindful living, resonated with the echoes of gratitude and the profound appreciation for the blessings they embraced. Each moment became an opportunity to acknowledge and celebrate the abundance in their lives.

Sarah, adorned with the grace of motherhood, led with a heart filled with gratitude—a beacon of appreciation, instilling in their child the value of thankfulness and the beauty of acknowledging life's blessings.

Meanwhile, Jackson, anchored in his paternal role, stood alongside Sarah—a partner in cultivating gratitude, ensuring their family embraced the ethos of appreciation in every aspect of their lives.

Together, they embraced the practice of gratitude—a symphony of shared thanks, a celebration of life's gifts, and a testament to the depth of their unity as they nurtured an environment steeped in appreciation and acknowledgment.

Their cultivation of gratitude became a cornerstone of their unity—a testament to their enduring love, dedication, and the profound appreciation that marked their journey as they nurtured their growing family.

Chapter Thirty-Nine: Weathering Storms

Amidst the tumultuous rhythms of their home, Sarah and Jackson found themselves navigating a phase marked by challenges—a testament to their resilience, unity, and unwavering commitment as they weathered the storms of parenthood.

Their home, once a sanctuary of peace, resonated with echoes of resilience and steadfastness. Each challenge they faced became an opportunity for growth, unity, and strengthening their bond as a family.

Sarah, adorned with the courage of motherhood, faced each trial with unwavering determination—a beacon of strength and perseverance, leading their family through the storms with unwavering grace.

Meanwhile, Jackson, grounded in his paternal role, stood by Sarah's side—a reliable ally, weathering the challenges together, ensuring their family remained resilient amidst the adversities.

Together, they navigated through the storms—a symphony of resilience, a demonstration of unity, and a testament to the depth of their commitment as they confronted and conquered the hurdles of parenthood.

Their shared experiences during this challenging phase became a testament to their unity—a reminder of their enduring love, resilience, and unwavering dedication as they stood strong, weathering the storms and emerging even stronger as a family.

Chapter Forty: The Everlasting Tapestry

In the serenity of their home, amidst the hushed whispers of a life well-lived, Sarah and Jackson found themselves at the culmination of a remarkable journey—a testament to their growth, unity, and the profound evolution they had experienced as parents.

Their home, a vessel of cherished memories, resonated with the echoes of a life interwoven with love, resilience, and an unbreakable bond forged through the passages of time. Each room whispered tales—a mosaic of laughter, tears, challenges, and triumphant moments—a vivid testament to the vibrant tapestry of their family life.

Sarah, adorned with the wisdom and grace of motherhood, stood as a beacon of nurturing strength—a testament to her unwavering dedication in shaping the lives entrusted to her care.

Meanwhile, Jackson, enriched by the depth of paternal love, stood as a steadfast guardian—a compass guiding their family through the ebb and flow of life, steadfast in his commitment to their shared journey.

Together, they had journeyed through the chapters—a symphony of shared experiences, endless devotion, and profound growth. Each moment etched a story—a legacy painted with the hues of love, dedication, and the enduring beauty of family bonds.

Their shared experiences had become a cherished heirloom—a testament to their unity, unwavering love, and the profound dedication that had illuminated every step of their exquisite voyage through parenthood.

As they stood hand in hand, gazing at the tapestry they had woven together, Sarah and Jackson embraced the beauty of their journey—a symphony of love, resilience, and unwavering commitment, celebrating the magnificence of their shared odyssey into parenthood.

THE END